OBSERVATIONS
ON
INSANITY.

OBSERVATIONS

ON

INSANITY.

WITH

PRACTICAL REMARKS ON THE DISEASE,

AND AN

ACCOUNT OF THE MORBID APPEARANCES ON DISSECTION.

By

JOHN HASLAM

"Of the uncertainties of our present state the most dreadful
and alarming is the uncertain continuance of reason."
Dr. Johnson's Rasselas.

TO THE
RIGHT WORSHIPFUL THE
PRESIDENT,
THE WORSHIPFUL THE
TREASURER, AND GOVERNORS
OF
BETHLEM-HOSPITAL.

MY LORDS AND GENTLEMEN,

The following Observations are respectfully submitted to YOUR notice, as the vigilant and humane Guardians of an *Institution* which performs much good to society, by diminishing the SEVEREST amongst human calamities,

By,
My Lords and Gentlemen,
Your very obedient and humble Servant,

The AUTHOR.

PREFACE.

AS the office I hold affords me abundant means of acquiring information on the subject of mental disorders, I should feel myself unworthy of that situation, were I to neglect any opportunity of accumulating such knowledge, or of communicating to the public any thing which might promise to be of advantage to mankind. The candid reader is therefore requested to accept this sentiment, as the best apology I can offer for the present production.

It has been somewhere observed, that in our own country more books on Insanity have been published than in any other; and, if the remark be just, it is certainly discouraging to him who proposes to add to their number. It must, however, be acknowledged, that we are but little indebted to those who have been most capable of affording us instruction; for, if we except the late Dr. John Monro's Reply to Dr. Battie's Treatise on Madness, there is no work on the subject of mental alienation which has been delivered on the authority of extensive observation and practice.

It is not intended to present the following sheets as a treatise, or compleat disquisition on the subject, but merely as remarks, which have occurred during the treatment of several hundred patients. As a knowledge of the structure, and functions of the body, have been held indispensably necessary in order to become acquainted with its diseases, and to a scientific mode of treating them; so it would appear, that he who proposes to write on Madness should be well informed concerning the powers and operations of the human mind: but the various and discordant opinions, which have prevailed in this department of knowledge, have led me to disentangle myself as quickly as possible from the perplexity of metaphysical mazes.

As some very erroneous notions have been entertained concerning the state of the brain, and more especially respecting its consistence in maniacal disorders, I have been induced to examine that viscus in those who have died insane, and have endeavoured with accuracy to report the appearances. It seemed proper to give some general history of these cases; perhaps the account which has been related of their erroneous opinions might have been spared, yet some friends whom I consulted expressed a wish that they had been more copiously detailed.

Of the difficulty of enumerating the remote causes of the disease I have been fully aware, and have mentioned but few, that I might be accused of the fewer mistakes. The prognosis contains some facts which, as far as I am informed, have not hitherto been made known, and appear to me of sufficient importance to be communicated to the public.

As it is my intention at some future period to attempt a more finished performance on the subject of Insanity, I shall feel grateful for any hints or observations, with which the kindness of professional gentlemen may supply me.

BETHLEM-HOSPITAL,
March 14, 1798.

OBSERVATIONS

ON

INSANITY.

CHAP. I.

READERS in general require a definition of the subject, which an author proposes to treat of; it is the duty therefore of every writer, to define, as clearly as he is able, that which he professes to elucidate.

A definition of a disease, should be a concentrated history, a selection of its prominent features and discriminative symptoms.

Of the definitions which have been given of this disease, some appear too contracted; and others not sufficiently precise.

1

Dr. Mead, after having treated largely upon the subject, concludes, "That this disease consists entirely in the strength of imagination." If the disease consisted entirely in the strength of imagination, the imagination ought to be equally strong upon all subjects, which upon accurate observation is not found to be the case. Had Dr. Mead stated, that, together with this increased strength of imagination, there existed an enfeebled state of the judgment, his definition would have been more correct. The strength, or increase of any power of the mind, cannot constitute a disease of it; strength of memory, has never been suspected to produce derangement of intellect; neither is it conceived, that great vigour of judgment can operate in any such manner; on the contrary it will readily be granted, that imbecility of memory must create confusion, by obstructing the action of the other powers of the mind; and that if the judgment be impaired, a man must necessarily speak, and generally act, in a very incorrect and ridiculous manner.

Dr. Ferriar, whom, to mention otherwise than as a man of genius, of learning, and of taste, would be unjust; has adopted the generally accepted division of Insanity, into Mania and Melancholy. In Mania, he conceives "false perception, and consequently confusion of ideas, to be a leading circumstance." The latter, he supposes to consist "in intensity of idea, which is a contrary state to false perception." From the observations I have been able to make respecting Mania, I have by no means been led to conclude, that false perception, is a leading circumstance in this disorder, and still less, that confusion of ideas must be the necessary consequence of false perception.

By perception, I understand, with Mr. Locke, the apprehension of sensations; and after a very diligent enquiry of patients who have recovered from the disease, and from an attentive observation of those labouring under it, I have not frequently found, that insane people perceive falsely, the objects which have been presented to them. It is true, that they all have false ideas, but this by no means infers, a defect of the power by which sensations are apprehended in the mind.

We find madmen equally deranged upon those ideas, which they have been long in the possession of, and on which the perception has not been recently exercised, as respecting those, which they have lately received: and we frequently find those who become suddenly mad, talk incoherently upon every subject, and consequently, upon many, on which the perception has not been exercised for a considerable time.

It is well known, that maniacs often suppose they have seen, and heard those things, which really did not exist at the time; but even this I should not explain by any disability, or error of the perception, since it is by no means the province of the perception to represent unreal existences to the mind. It must therefore be sought elsewhere, probably in the senses, or in the imagination.

I have known eight cases of patients, who insisted that they had seen the devil. It might be urged, that in these instances, the perception was vitiated; but it must be observed, that there could be no perception of that, which was not present and existing at the time. Upon desiring these patients to describe what they had seen, they all represented him as a big, black man, with a long tail, cloven feet, and sharp talons, such as is seen pictured in books. A proof that the idea was revived in the mind from some former impressions. One of these patients however carried the matter a little further, as she solemnly declared, she heard him break the iron chain with which God had confined him, and saw him pass fleetly by her window, with a truss of straw upon his shoulder.

It must be acknowledged, that in the soundest state of our faculties we sometimes perceive things which do not exist. If the middle finger be crossed over the forefinger, and a single pea be rolled under their extremities, we have the perception of *two*. By immersing one hand into warm, the other into cold water, and afterwards suddenly plunging them both into the same fluid, of a medium temperature, we shall derive the sensations of heat, and cold from the same water, at the same time.

The power, by which the mind perceives its own creations and combinations is perhaps the same, as that by which it perceives the impressions on the senses from external objects. We possess the faculty of raising up of objects in the mind which we had seen before, and of prospects, on which we had formerly dwelt, with admiration and delight; and in the coolest state of our understanding we can even conceive that they lie before us. If the power which awakens these remembrances in a healthy state of intellect, should stir up distorted combinations in disease, they must necessarily be perceived; but their apprehension, by no means appears to imply a vitiated state of the faculty by which they are perceived. In fact, that which is represented to the mind, either by a defect or deception of the senses, or by the imagination, if it be sufficiently forcible and enduring, must necessarily be perceived.

That "confusion of ideas" should be the necessary consequence of false perception, is very difficult to admit. Perhaps much may depend, in the discussion of this point, on the various acceptations in which confusion of ideas may be understood.

It has often been observed that madmen, will frequently reason correctly from false premises, and the observation is certainly true: we have indeed occasion to notice the same thing in those of the soundest minds. It is very possible for the perception to be deceived in the occurrence of a thing, which, although it did not actually happen, yet was likely to take place; and which had frequently occurred before. The reception of this as a truth in the mind, if the power of deducing from it the proper inferences existed, could neither create confusion, nor irregularity of ideas.

Melancholy, the other form in which this disease is supposed to exist, is made by Dr. Ferriar to consist in "intensity of idea." I shall shortly have an opportunity, in the definition I propose to give, of attempting to prove, that this division of Insanity, is neither natural nor just, upon the ground that the derangement is equally complete in both forms of the disease. We ought to attend more to the state of the intellect, than to the passions which accompany the disorder.

By intensity of idea, I presume is meant, that the mind is more strongly fixed on, or more frequently recurs to, a certain set of ideas, than when it is in a healthy state. But this definition applies equally to mania, for we every day see the most furious maniacs suddenly sink into a profound melancholy; and the most depressed, and miserable objects, become violent and raving. We have patients in Bethlem Hospital, whose lives are divided between furious, and melancholic paroxisms; and who, under both states, retain the same set of ideas.

Insanity may, in my opinion, be defined to be *an incorrect association of familiar ideas, which is independent of the prejudices of education, and is always accompanied with implicit belief, and generally with either violent or depressing passions.* It appears to me necessary, that the ideas incorrectly associated, should be *familiar*, because we can hardly be said to have our ideas deranged upon subjects, concerning which we have little or no information. A peasant, who had heard that superior comforts of life, with fewer exertions, were to be obtained by emigrating to America, might saddle his beast with an intention of riding thither on horse-back, without any other imputation than that of ignorance; but if an old and experienced navigator, were to propose a similar mode of conveyance, I should have little hesitation in concluding him insane.

Respecting the prejudices of education, it may be observed, that in our childhood, and before we are able to form a true, and accurate judgment of things, we have impressed upon our minds, a number of ideas which are ridiculous; but which were the received opinions of the place in which we then lived, and of the people who inculcated them; such is the belief in the powers of witchcraft, and in ghosts, and superstitions of every denomination, which grasp strongly upon the mind and seduce its credulity. There are many honest men in this kingdom who would not sleep quietly, if a vessel filled with quicksilver were to be brought into their houses; they would perhaps feel alarmed for the chastity of their wives and daughters; and this, because they had been taught to consider that many strange and unaccountable properties are attached to that metal. If a lecturer on chemistry were to exhibit the same fears, there could be no doubt that he laboured under a disorder of intellect, because the properties of mercury would be known to him, and his alarms would arise from incorrectly associating ideas of danger, with a substance, which in that state is innoxious, and whose properties come within the sphere of his knowledge.

As the terms Mania, and Melancholy, are in general use, and serve to distinguish the forms under which insanity is exhibited, there can be no objection to retain them; but I would strongly oppose their being considered as opposite diseases. In both, the association of ideas is equally incorrect, and they appear to differ only, from the different passions which accompany them. On dissection, the state of the brain does not shew any appearances peculiar to melancholy; nor is the treatment which I have observed most successful, different from that which is employed in Mania.

CHAP. II.

SYMPTOMS OF THE DISEASE.

With most authors, this part of the subject has occupied the greatest share of their labour and attention: they have generally descended to minute particularities and studied discriminations. Distinctions have been created, rather from the peculiar turn of the patients propensities and discourse, than from any marked difference, in the varieties, and species of the disorder: and it has been customary to ornament this part of the work with copious citations from poetical writers. As my plan extends only to a description of that which I have observed, I shall neither amplify, nor embellish my volume by quotations.

In most public hospitals, the first attack of diseases is seldom to be observed; and it might naturally be supposed, that there existed in Bethlem, similar impediments to an accurate knowledge of madness. It is true, that all who are admitted into it have been a greater, or less time afflicted with the complaint; yet from the occasional relapses to which insane persons are subject, we have frequent and sufficient opportunities of observing the beginning, and tracing the progress of this disease.

Among the incurables, there are some who have intervals of perfect soundness of mind; but who are subject to relapses, which would render it improper, and even dangerous, to trust them at large in society: and with those who are upon the curable list, a recurrence of the malady very frequently takes place. Upon these occasions, there is ample scope for observing the first attack of the disease.

To enumerate every symptom would be descending to useless minutiæ, I shall therefore content myself with describing the more general appearances.

They first become uneasy, are incapable of confining their attention, and neglect any employment to which they have been accustomed; they get but little sleep, they are loquacious, and disposed to harangue, and decide promptly, and positively upon every subject that may be started. Soon after, they are divested of all restraint in the declaration of their opinions of those, with whom they are acquainted. Their friendships are expressed with fervency and extravagance; their enmities with intolerance and disgust. They now become impatient of contradiction, and scorn reproof. For supposed injuries, they are inclined to quarrel, and fight with those about them. They have all the appearance of persons inebriated, and people unacquainted with the symptoms of approaching mania, generally suppose them to be in a state of intoxication. At length suspicion creeps in upon the mind, they are aware of plots which had never been contrived, and detect motives that were never entertained. At last, the succession of ideas is too rapid to be examined; the mind becomes crouded with thoughts, and indiscriminately jumbles them together.

Those under the influence of the depressing passions, will exhibit a different train of symptoms. The countenance, wears an anxious and gloomy aspect. They retire from the company of those with whom they had formerly associated, seclude themselves in obscure places, or lie in bed the greatest part of their time. They next become fearful, and, when irregular combinations of ideas have taken place, conceive a thousand fancies: often recur to some former immoral act which they have committed, or imagine themselves guilty of crimes which they never perpetrated; believe that God has abandoned them, and with trembling, await his punishment. Frequently they become desperate, and endeavour by their own hands to terminate an existence, which appears to be an afflicting and hateful incumbrance.

The sound mind seems to consist in a harmonized association of its different powers, and is so constituted, that a defect, in any one, produces irregularity, and, most commonly, derangement of the whole. The different forms therefore under which we see this disease, might not, perhaps, be improperly arranged according to the powers which are chiefly affected.

I have before remarked, that the increased vigor of any mental faculty cannot constitute intellectual disease. If the memory of a person were so retentive, that he could re-assemble the whole of what he had heard, read, and thought, such a man, even with a moderate understanding, would pass through life with reputation and utility. Suppose another to possess a judgment, so discriminating and correct, that he could ascertain precisely, the just weight of every argument; this man would be a splendid ornament to human society. Let the imagination of a third, create images and scenes, which mankind should ever view with rapture and astonishment, such a phænomenon would bring Shakespear to our recollection.

If in a chain of ideas, a number of the links are broken, the mind cannot possess any accurate information. When patients of this description are asked a question, they appear as if awakened from a sound sleep; they are searching, they know not where, for the proper materials of an answer, and, in the painful, and fruitless efforts of recollection, generally lose sight of the question itself.

In persons of sound mind, as well as in maniacs, the memory is the first power which decays, and there is something remarkable in the manner of its decline. The transactions of the latter part of life are feebly recollected, whilst the scenes of youth, and of manhood, remain more strongly impressed. To many conversations of the old incurable patients to which I have listened, the topic has always turned upon the scenes of early days. In many cases, where the faculties of the mind have been injured by intemperance, the same withering of the recollection may be observed. It may perhaps arise, from the mind at an early period of life being most susceptible and retentive of impressions, and from a greater disposition to be pleased with the objects which are presented: whereas, the cold caution, and fastidiousness with which age surveys the prospects of life, joined to the dulness of the senses, and the slight curiosity which prevails, will, in some degree, explain the difficulty, or rather impossibility, of recalling the history of later transactions.

Insane people who have been good scholars, after a long confinement lose, in a wonderful degree, the correctness of orthography; when they write, above half the words are generally mis-spelt — they are written according to the pronunciation. It shews how treacherous the memory is without reinforcement. The same necessity of a constant recruit and frequent review of our ideas, satisfactorily explains, why a number of patients lapse nearly into a state of ideotism. These have, for some years, been the silent and gloomy inhabitants of the Hospital, who have avoided conversation, and sought solitude; consequently have acquired no new ideas, and time has effaced the impression of those formerly stamped upon the mind. Mr. Locke well observes, "that there seems to be a constant decay of all our ideas, even of those which are struck deepest, and in minds the most retentive; so that if they be not sometimes renewed, by repeated exercise of the senses, or reflection on those kind of objects, which at first occasioned them; the print wears out, and at last there remains nothing to be seen."

As it has been attempted to explain, how an imbecility or loss of memory will obstruct the operation of the other powers of the mind: the next object is to shew, how necessarily our ideas must be disarranged where the determination on their comparison is wrong, or where the mind determines, or judges, with little previous examination or comparison. An example or two will illustrate this more satisfactorily than any length of reasoning. I remember a patient who conceived, that, although dead men told no tales, yet their feeling was very acute. This assumed principle he extended to inferior animals, and refused to eat meat, because he could not endure to be nourished at the expence of the cruel sufferings, which beef steaks necessarily underwent in their cookery. Another madman, who pretended to extraordinary skill in surgery, contrived to steal the wooden leg of an insane patient, and laid upon it for a considerable time, with a firm belief of hatching it into a limb of flesh and blood.

If a man shall form such ideas, and conceive them to be true, either from a defect in the power of his judgment, or without any comparison or examination shall infer them to be so, such defect will afford a sufficient source of derangement.

Some who have perfectly recovered from this disease, and who are persons of good understanding and liberal education, describe the state they were in as resembling a dream; and, when they have been told how long they were disordered, have been astonished that the time passed so rapidly away. Others speak of their disorder as accompanied with great hurry and confusion of mind, where the succession of ideas is so rapid and evanescent, that when they have endeavoured to arrest or contemplate any particular thoughts, they have been carried away by the tide, which was rolling after them.

All patients have not the same degree of memory of what has passed during the time they were disordered: but for the most part they recollect those ideas which were transmitted through the medium of the senses, better than the combinations of their own minds. I have frequently remarked that, when they were unable to give any account of the peculiar opinions which they had indulged during a raving paroxysm of long continuance, they well remembered any coercion which had been used, or any kindness which had been shewn them.

Insane people are said to be generally worse in the morning; in some cases they certainly are so, but perhaps not so frequently as has been supposed. In many instances (and, as far as I have observed) in the beginning of the disease they are more violent in the evening, and continue so the greatest part of the night. It is however a certain fact, that the majority of patients of this description have their symptoms aggravated, by being placed in a recumbent posture.

They seem themselves to avoid the horizontal position as much as possible when they are in a raving state: and when so confined that they cannot be erect, they will keep themselves seated upon the breech.

Many of those who are violently disordered will continue particular actions for a considerable time: some are heard to gingle the chain, with which they are confined, for hours without intermission; others, who are secured in an erect posture, will beat the ground with their feet the greatest part of the day. Upon enquiry of such patients, after they have recovered, they have assured me, that these actions afforded them considerable relief. We often surprize persons who are free from intellectual disease in many strange and ridiculous movements, particularly if their minds be intently occupied:—this does not appear to be the effect of habit, but of a particular state of mind.

Madmen do not always continue in the same furious or depressed states: the maniacal paroxysm abates of its violence, and some beams of hope occasionally cheer the despondency of the melancholick patients. We have some unfortunate persons who are obliged to be secured the greatest part of their time, but who now and then become calm, and to a certain degree rational: upon such occasions, they are allowed a greater range, and are permitted to associate with the others. In some instances, the degree of rationality is more considerable; they conduct themselves with propriety, and in a short conversation will appear sensible and coherent. Such remission, has been generally termed a *lucid interval*.

When medical men are called upon to attend a commission of lunacy, they are always asked, whether the patient has had a *lucid interval*? A term of such latitude as *interval* requires to be explained in the most perspicuous and accurate manner. In common language it is made to signify, both a moment and a number of years, consequently it does not comprize any stated time. The term *lucid interval* is therefore relative. I should define a *lucid interval* to be *a complete recovery of the patient's intellects, ascertained by repeated examinations of his conversation, and by constant observation of his conduct, for a time sufficient to enable the superintendant to form a correct judgment*. Unthinking people are frequently led to conclude that, if during a conversation of a few minutes, a person under confinement shall betray nothing absurd or incorrect, he is well, and often remonstrate on the injustice of secluding him from the world. Even in common society, there are many persons whom we never suspect from a few trifling topics of discourse to be shallow minded; but, if we start a subject, and wish to discuss it through all it's ramifications and dependances we find them incapable of pursuing a connected chain of reasoning. In the same manner, insane people will often, for a short time, conduct themselves, both in conversation and behaviour, with such propriety, that they appear to have the just exercise and direction of their faculties; but let the examiner protract the discourse, until the favourite subject shall have got afloat in the madman's brain, and he will be convinced of the hastiness of his decision. To those unaccustomed to insane people, a few coherent sentences, or rational answers would indicate a lucid interval, because they discover no madness; but he who is in possession of the peculiar turn of the patient's thoughts, might lead him to disclose them, or by a continuance of the conversation they would spontaneously break forth. A beautiful illustration of this is contained in the Rasselas of Dr. Johnson: where the astronomer is admired as a person of sound intellect and great acquirements by Imlac, who is himself a philosopher, and a man of the world. His intercourse with the astronomer is frequent; and he always finds in his society information and delight. At length he receives Imlac into the most unbounded confidence, and imparts to him the momentous secret. "Hear Imlac what thou wilt not without difficulty credit. I have possessed for five years the regulation of weather, and the distribution of the seasons. The sun has listened to my dictates, and passed from tropic to tropic by my direction. The clouds at my call have poured their waters, and the Nile has overflowed at my command. I have restrained the rage of the Dog-star, and mitigated the fervours of the Crab. The winds alone of all the elemental powers have hitherto refused my authority, and multitudes have perished by equinoctial tempests, which I found myself unable to prohibit or restrain. I have administered this great office with exact justice, and made to the different nations of the Earth an impartial dividend of rain and sunshine. What must have been the misery of half the globe, if I had limited the clouds to particular regions, or confined the sun to either side of the equator?"

A real case came under my observation a few months ago, and which is equally apposite to the subject. A young man had become insane from habitual intoxication, and during the violence of his complaint had attempted to destroy himself. Under a supposed imputation of having unnatural dispositions he had amputated his penis, with a view of precluding any future insinuations of that nature. For many months after he was admitted into the hospital, he continued in a state which obliged him to be strictly confined, as he constantly meditated his own destruction. On a sudden he became apparently well, was highly sensible of the delusion under which he had laboured, and conversed as any other person upon the ordinary topics of discourse. There was, however, something in the reserve of his manner, and peculiarity of his look, which persuaded me that he was not well, although no incoherence of ideas could be detected in his conversation. I had observed him for some days to walk rather lame, and once or twice had noticed him sitting with his shoes off, rubbing his feet. On enquiring into the motives of his doing so, he replied, that his feet were blistered, and wished that some remedy might be applied to remove the vesications. When I requested to look at his feet, he declined it and prevaricated, saying, that they were only tender and uncomfortable. In a few days afterwards, he assured me they were perfectly well. The next evening I observed him, unperceived, still rubbing his feet, and then peremptorily insisted on examining them. They were quite free from any disorder. He now told me with some embarrassment, that he wished much for a confidential friend, to whom he might impart a secret of importance. Upon assuring him that he might trust me, he said, that the boards on which he walked, (the second story) were heated by subterraneous fires, under the direction of invisible and malicious agents, whose intentions, he was well convinced, were to consume him by degrees.

From these considerations I am inclined to think, that a *lucid interval* includes all the circumstances which I have enumerated in my definition of it. If the person who is to examine the state of the patient's mind be unacquainted with his peculiar opinions, he may be easily deceived, because, wanting this information, he will have no clue to direct his enquiries, and madmen do not always, nor immediately intrude their incoherent notions into notice. They have sometimes such a high degree of controul over their minds, that when they have any particular purpose to carry, they will affect to renounce those opinions which shall have been judged inconsistent: and it is well known that they have often dissembled their resentment, until a favourable opportunity has occurred of gratifying their revenge.

Among the bodily particularities which mark this disease, may be observed the protruded, and oftentimes glistening eye, and a peculiar cast of countenance which, however, cannot be described. In some, an appearance takes place which has not hitherto been noticed by Authors. This is a relaxation of the integuments of the cranium, by means of which they may be wrinkled, or rather gathered up by the hand to a considerable degree. It is generally most remarkable on the posterior part of the scalp; as far as my enquiries have reached, it does not take place in the beginning of the disease, but after a raving paroxysm of some continuance. It has been frequently accompanied with contraction of the iris.

On the suggestion of a medical gentleman, I was induced to ascertain the prevailing complexion and colour of the hair in insane patients. Out of 265 who were examined, 205 were of a swarthy complection, with dark, or black hair; the remaining 60 were of a fair skin, and light, brown, or red haired. What connection this proportion may have with the complection and colour of the hair of the people of this country in general, and what alterations may have been produced by age or residence in other climates, I am totally uninformed.

Of the power which maniacs possess of resisting cold the belief is general, and the histories which are on record are truly wonderful. It is not my wish to disbelieve, nor my intention to dispute them; it is proper, however, to state, that the patients in Bethlem hospital possess no such exemption from the effects of severe cold. They are particularly subject to mortifications of the feet; and this fact is so well established from former accidents, that there is an express order of the house, that every patient, under strict confinement, shall have his feet examined morning and evening by the keeper, and also have them constantly wrapped in flannel; and those who are permitted to go about are always to be found as near to the fire as they can get, during the winter season.

Having thus given a general account of the symptoms which I have observed to occur most commonly in persons affected with madness, I shall now lay before my readers a history of all the appearances which I have noticed on opening the heads of several maniacs, who have died in Bethlem Hospital.

CASE I.

J. H. a man twenty-eight years of age, was admitted a patient in May 1795. He had been disordered for about two months before he came into the hospital. No particular cause was stated to have brought on the complaint. It was most probably an hereditary affection, as his father had been several times insane and confined in our hospital. During the time he was in the house, he was in a very low and melancholic state; shewed an aversion to food, and said he was resolved to die. His obstinacy in refusing all nourishment was very great, and it was with much difficulty forced upon him. He continued in this state, but became daily weaker and more emaciated until August 1st when he died. Upon opening the head, the pericranium was found loosely adherent to the scull. The bones of the cranium were thick. The pia mater was loaded with blood, and the medullary substance, when cut into, was full of bloody points. The pineal gland contained a large quantity of gritty matter[1]. The consistence of the brain was natural; he was opened twenty-four hours after death.

CASE II.

J. W. was a man of sixty-two years of age, who had been many years in the house as an incurable patient, but with the other parts of whose history I am totally unacquainted. He appeared to be a quiet and inoffensive person, who found amusement in his own thoughts, and seldom joined in any conversation with the other patients: for some months he had been troubled with a cough, attended with copious expectoration, which very much reduced him; dropsical symptoms followed these complaints. He became every day weaker, and on July 10th, 1795, died. He was opened eighteen hours after death. The pericranium adhered loosely to the scull; the bones of the cranium were unusually thin. There were slight opacities in many parts of the tunica arachnoides; in the ventricles about four ounces of water were contained — some large hydatids were discovered on the plexus choroides of the right side. The consistence of the brain was natural.

CASE III.

G. H. a man twenty-six years of age, was received into the hospital July 18th, 1795. It was stated that he had been disordered six weeks previous to his admission, and that he had never had any former attack. He had been a drummer with a recruiting party, and had been for some time in the habit of constant intoxication, which was assigned as the cause of his insanity. He continued in a violent and raving state about a month, during the whole of which time he got little or no sleep. He had no knowledge of his situation but supposed himself with the regiment, and was frequently under great anxiety and alarm for the loss of his drum, which he imagined had been stolen and sold. The medicines which were given to him he conceived were spirituous liquors, and swallowed them with avidity. At the expiration of a month, he was very weak and reduced; his legs became œdematous—his pupils were much diminished. He now believed himself a child, called upon the people about him as his playfellows, and appeared to recall the scenes of early life with facility and correctness. Within a few days of his decease he only muttered to himself. August 26th, he died. He was opened six hours after death. The pericranium was loosely adherent. The tunica arachnoides had generally lost its transparency, and was considerably thickened. The veins of the pia mater were loaded with blood, and in many places seemed to contain air. There was a considerable quantity of water between the membranes, and as nearly as could be ascertained about four ounces in the ventricles, in the cavity of which, the veins appeared remarkably turgid. The consistence of the brain was more than usually firm.

CASE IV.

E. M. a woman, aged sixty, was admitted into the house, August 8th, 1795; she had been disordered five months; the cause assigned was extreme grief, in consequence of the loss of her only daughter. She was very miserable and restless; conceived she had been accused of some horrid crime, for which she apprehended she should be burned alive. When any persons entered her room she supposed them officers of justice, who were about to drag her to some cruel punishment. She was frequently violent, and would strike and bite those who came near her. Upon the idea that she should shortly be put to death, she refused all sustenance; and it became necessary to force her to take it. In this state she continued, growing daily weaker and more emaciated, until October 3d, when she died.

Upon opening the head there was a copious determination of blood to the whole contents of the cranium. The pia mater was considerably inflamed; there was not any water either in the ventricles or between the membranes. The brain was particularly soft. She was opened thirty hours after death.

CASE V.

W. P. a young man aged twenty-five, was admitted into the hospital September 26, 1795. He had been disordered five months, and had experienced a similar attack six years before. The disease was brought on by excessive drinking. He was in a very furious state, in consequence of which he was constantly confined. He got little or no sleep—during the greater part of the night he was singing, or swearing, or holding conversations with persons he imagined to be about him: sometimes he would rattle the chain with which he was confined for several hours together, and tore every thing to pieces within his reach. In the beginning of November the violence of his disorder subsided for two or three days, but afterwards returned; and on the 10th he died compleatly exhausted by his exertions.—Upon opening the head the pericranium was found firmly attached; the pia mater was inflamed, though not to any very considerable degree; the tunica arachnoides in some places was slightly shot with blood; the membranes of the brain, and its convolutions when these were removed, were of a brown, or brownish straw colour. There was no water in any of the cavities of the brain, nor any particular congestion of blood in its substance—the consistence of which was natural. He was opened twenty hours after death.

CASE VI.

B. H. was an incurable patient, who had been confined in the house from the year 1788, and for some years before that time in a private madhouse. He was about sixty years of age—had formerly been in the habit of intoxicating himself. His character was strongly marked by pride, irascibility, and malevolence. During the four last years of his life he was confined for attempting to commit some violence on one of the officers of the house. After this he was seldom heard to speak; yet he manifested his evil disposition by every species of dumb insult. Latterly he grew suspicious, and would sometimes tell the keeper that his victuals were poisoned. About the beginning of December he was taken ill with a cough, attended with copious expectoration. Being then asked respecting his complaints, he said he had a violent pain across the stomach, which arose from his navel string at his birth having been tied too short. He never spoke afterwards, though frequently importuned to describe his complaints. He died December 24, 1795.

Upon dividing the integuments of the head, the pericranium was found scarcely to adhere to the scull. On the right parietal bone there was a large blotch, as if the bone had been inflamed: there were others on different parts of the bone, but considerably smaller. The glandulæ Pacchioni were uncommonly large: the tunica arachnoides in many places wanted the natural transparency of that membrane: there was a large determination of blood to the substance of the brain: the ventricles contained about three ounces of water; the consistence of the brain was natural. He was opened two days after death.

CASE VII.

A. M. a woman aged twenty-seven, was admitted into the hospital August 15, 1795; she had then been eleven weeks disordered. Religious enthusiasm, and a too frequent attendance on conventicles, were stated to have occasioned her complaint. She was in a very miserable and unhappy condition, and terrified by the most alarming apprehensions for the salvation of her soul. Towards the latter end of September she appeared in a convalescent state, and continued tolerably well until the middle of November, when she began to relapse.

The return of her disorder commenced with loss of sleep. She alternately sang, and cried the greatest part of the night. She conceived her inside full of the most loathsome vermin, and often felt the sensation as if they were crawling into her throat. She was suddenly seized with a strong and unconquerable determination to destroy herself; became very sensible of her malady, and said, that God had inflicted this punishment on her, from having (at some former part of her life) said the Lord's Prayer backwards. She continued some time in a restless and forlorn state; at one moment expecting the devil to seize upon her and tear her to pieces; in the next, wondering that she was not instigated to commit violence on the persons about her. On January 12, 1796, she died suddenly. She was opened twelve hours after death. The thoracic and abdominal viscera were perfectly healthy.

Upon examining the contents of the cranium, the pia mater was considerably inflamed, and an extravasated blotch, about the size of a shilling, was seen upon that membrane, near the middle of the right lobe of the cerebrum. There was no water between the membranes, nor in the ventricles, but a general determination of blood to the contents of the cranium. The medullary substance when cut into was full of bloody points. The consistence of the brain was natural.

CASE VIII.

M. W. a very tall and thin woman, forty-four years of age, was admitted into the hospital September 19, 1795. Her disorder was of six months standing, and eight years before she had also had an attack of this disease. The cause assigned to have brought it on, the last time, was the loss of some property, the disease having shortly followed that circumstance. The constant tenor of her discourse was, that she should live but a short time. She seemed anxiously to wish for her dissolution, but had no thoughts of accomplishing her own destruction. In the course of a few weeks she began to imagine, that some malevolent person had given her mercury with an intention to destroy her. She was constantly shewing her teeth, which had decayed naturally, as if this effect had been produced by that medicine: at last she insisted, that mercurial preparations were mingled in the food and medicines which were administered to her. Her appetite was voracious notwithstanding this belief. She had a continual thirst, and drank very large quantities of cold water.

On January 14, 1796, she had an apoplectic fit, well marked by stertor, loss of voluntary motion, and insensibility to stimuli. On the following day she died. She was opened two days after death. There was a remarkable accumulation of blood in the veins of the dura and pia mater; the substance of the brain was loaded with blood. When the medullary substance was cut into blood oozed from it; and upon squeezing it a greater quantity could be forced out. On the pia mater covering the right lobe of the cerebrum, were some slight extravasations of blood. The ventricles contained no water; on the plexus choroides were some vesicles of the size of coriander-seeds, filled with a yellow fluid. The pericranium adhered firmly to the scull. The consistence of the brain was firmer than usual.

CASE IX.

E. D. a woman aged thirty-six, was admitted into the hospital February 20, 1795: she had then been disordered four months. Her insanity came on a few days after having been delivered. She had also laboured under a similar attack seven years before, which, like the present, supervened upon the birth of a child. Under the impression that she ought to be hanged, she destroyed her infant, with the view of meeting with that punishment. When she came into the house, she was very sensible of the crime she had committed, and felt the most poignant affliction for the act. For about a month she continued to amend: after which time she became more thoughtful, and frequently spoke about the child: great anxiety and restlessness succeeded. In this state she remained until April 23, when her tongue became thickly furred, the skin parched, her eyes inflamed and glassy, and her pulse quick. She now talked incoherently; and, towards the evening, merely muttered to herself. She died on the following day comatose.

She was opened about twenty-four hours after death. The scull was thick, the pericranium scarcely adhered to the bone, the dura mater was also but slightly attached to its internal surface. There was a large quantity of water between the dura mater and tunica arachnoidea; this latter membrane was much thickened, and was of a milky white appearance. Between the tunica arachnoidea and pia mater, there was a considerable accumulation of water. The veins of the pia mater were particularly turgid. About three ounces of water were contained in the lateral ventricles: the veins of the membrane lining these cavities were remarkably large and turgid with blood. When the medullary substance of the cerebrum and cerebellum was cut into, there appeared a great number of bloody points. The brain was of its natural consistence.

CASE X.

C. M. a man forty years of age, was admitted into the hospital Dec. 26, 1795. It was stated, that he had been disordered two months previous to his having been received as a patient. His friends were unacquainted with any cause, which was likely to have induced the complaint. During the time he was in the house he seemed sulky, or rather stupid. He never asked any questions, and if spoken to, either replied shortly, or turned away without giving any answer. He appeared to take little notice of any thing which was going forward, and if told to do any little office, generally forgot what he was going about, before he had advanced half a dozen steps. He remained in this state until the beginning of May, 1796, when his legs became œdematous, and his abdomen swollen. He grew very feeble and helpless, and died rather suddenly

May 19th. He was opened about forty-eight hours after death. The pericranium and dura mater adhered firmly to the scull; in many places there was an opake whiteness of the tunica arachnoides. About four ounces of water were found in the ventricles. The plexus choroides were uncommonly pale. The medullary substance, afforded hardly any bloody points when cut into. The consistence of the brain I cannot describe better than by saying, it was doughy.

CASE XI.

S. M. a man thirty-six years of age, was admitted as an incurable patient in the year 1790. Of the former history of his complaint I have no information. As his habits, which frequently came under my observation, were of a singular nature, it may not here be improper to relate them. Having at some period of his confinement been mischievously disposed, and, in consequence, put under coercion, he never afterwards found himself comfortable when at liberty. When he rose in the morning he went immediately to the room where he was usually confined, and placed himself in a particular corner, until the keeper came to secure him. If he found any other patient had pre-occupied his situation, he became very outrageous, and generally forced them to leave it. When he had been confined, for which he appeared anxious, as he bore any delay with little temper, he employed himself throughout the remainder of the day, by tramping or shuffling his feet. He was constantly muttering to himself, of which scarcely one word in a sentence was intelligible. When an audible expression escaped him it was commonly an imprecation. If a stranger visited him, he always asked for tobacco, but seldom repeated his solicitation. He devoured his food with avidity, and always muttered as he ate.

In the month of July, 1796, he was seized with a diarrhœa, which afterwards terminated in dysentery. This continued, notwithstanding the employment of every medicine usually given in such a case, until his death, which took place on September 23, of the same year. He was opened twelve hours after death. The scull was unusually thin; the glandulæ Pacchioni were large and numerous: there was a very general determination of blood to the brain: the medullary substance, when cut, shewed an abundance of bloody points: the lateral ventricles contained about four ounces of water: the consistence of the brain was natural.

CASE XII.

E. R. was a woman, to all appearance about eighty years of age, but of whose history, before she came into the hospital, it has not been in my power to acquire any satisfactory intelligence. She was an incurable patient, and had been admitted on that establishment in February 1782.

During the time I had an opportunity of observing her, she continued in the same state: she appeared feeble and childish. During the course of the day, she sat in a particular part of the common-room, from which she never stirred. Her appetite was tolerably good, but it was requisite to feed her. Except she was particularly urged to speak she never talked. As the summer declined she grew weaker, and died October 19, 1796, apparently worn out. She was opened two days after death. The scull was particularly thin; the pericranium adhered firmly to the bone, and the scull-cap was with difficulty separated from the dura mater. There was a very large quantity of water between the membranes of the brain: the glandulæ Pacchioni were uncommonly large: the tunica arachnoidea was in many places blotched and streaked with opacities: when the medullary substance of the brain was cut into, it was every where bloody; and blood could be pressed from it, as from a sponge. There were some large hydatids on the plexus choroides: in the ventricles about a tea spoonful of water was observed: the consistence of the brain was particularly firm, but it could not be called elastic. There were no symptoms of general dropsy.

CASE XIII.

J. D. a man thirty-five years of age, was admitted into the hospital in October 1796. He was a person of good education, and had been regularly brought up to medicine, which he had practised in this town for several years. It was stated by his friends, that, about two years before, he had suffered a similar attack, which continued six months: but it appears from the observations of some medical persons, that he never perfectly recovered from it, although he returned to the exercise of his profession. A laborious attention to business, and great apprehensions of the want of success, were assigned as causes of his malady. In the beginning of the year 1796 the disease recurred, and became so violent that it was necessary to confine him.

At the time he was received into Bethlem hospital, he was in an unquiet state, got little or no sleep, and was constantly speaking loudly: in general he was worse towards evening. He appeared little sensible of external objects: his exclamations were of the most incoherent nature.

During the time he was a patient he was thrice cupped on the scalp. After each operation, he became rational to a certain degree; but these intervals were of a short continuance, as he relapsed in the course of a few hours. The scalp, particularly at the posterior part of the head, was so loose that a considerable quantity of it could be gathered up by the hand[2]. The violence of his exertions at last exhausted him, and, on December 11, he died. He was opened about twenty-four hours after death. There was a large quantity of water between the dura mater and tunica arachnoidea, and also between this latter membrane and the pia mater. The arachnoid membrane was thickened and opake; the vessels of the pia mater were loaded with blood: when the medullary substance was cut into, it was very abundant in bloody points: about three ounces of water were contained in the lateral ventricles: the plexus choroides were remarkably turgid with blood: a quantity of water was found in the theca vertebralis: the consistence of the brain was natural.

CASE XIV.

J. C. a man aged sixty-one, was admitted into the hospital September 17, 1796. It was stated that he had been disordered ten months. He had for thirty years kept a public house, and had for some time been in the habit of getting intoxicated. His memory was considerably impaired: circumstances were so feebly impressed on his mind, that he was unable to give any account of the preceding day. He appeared perfectly reconciled to his situation, and conducted himself with order and propriety. As he seldom spoke but when interrogated, it was not possible to collect his opinions. In this quiet state he continued about two months, when he became more thoughtful and abstracted, walked about with a quick step, and frequently started, as if suddenly interrupted. He was next seized with trembling, appeared anxious to be released from his confinement: conceived at one time that his house was filled with company; at another that different people had gone off without paying him, and that he should be arrested for sums of money which he owed. Under this constant alarm and disquietude he continued about a week, when he became sullen and refused his food. When importuned to take nourishment, he said it was ridiculous to offer it to him, as he had no mouth to eat it: though forced to take it, he continued in the same opinion; and when food was put into his mouth, insisted that a wound had been made in his throat, in order to force it into his stomach. The next day he complained of violent pain in his head, and in a few minutes afterwards died. He was opened twelve hours after death. There was a large quantity of water between the tunica arachnoidea and pia mater; the latter membrane was much suffused with blood, and many of its vessels were considerably enlarged: the lateral ventricles contained at least six ounces of water: the brain was very firm.

CASE XV.

J. A. a man forty-two years of age, was first admitted into the house on June 27, 1795. His disease came on suddenly whilst he was working in a garden, on a very hot day, without any covering to his head. He had some years before travelled with a gentleman over a great part of Europe: his ideas ran particularly on what he had seen abroad; sometimes he conceived himself the king of Denmark, at other times the king of France. Although naturally dull and wanting common education, he professed himself a master of all the dead and living languages; but his most intimate acquaintance was with the old French; and he was persuaded he had some faint recollection of coming over to this country with William the Conqueror. His temper was very irritable, and he was disposed to quarrel with every body about him. After he had continued ten months in the hospital, he became tranquil, relinquished his absurdities, and was discharged well in June 1796. He went into the country with his wife to settle some domestic affairs, and in about six weeks afterwards relapsed. He was readmitted into the hospital August 13th.

He now evidently had a paralytic affection, his speech was inarticulate, and his mouth drawn aside. He shortly became stupid, his legs swelled and afterwards ulcerated; at length his appetite failed him; he became emaciated, and died December 27th, of the same year. The head was opened twenty hours after death. There was a greater quantity of water between the different membranes of the brain than has ever occurred to me. The tunica arachnoidea was generally opake and very much thickened: the pia mater was loaded with blood, and the veins of that membrane were particularly enlarged. On the fore-part of the right hemisphere of the brain, when stripped of its membranes, there was a blotch, of a brown colour, several shades darker than the rest of the cortical substance: the ventricles were much enlarged, and contained, by estimation, at least six ounces of water. The veins in these cavities were particularly turgid. The consistence of the brain was firmer than usual.

CASE XVI.

J. H. a man aged forty-two, was admitted into the house on April 12, 1794. He had then been disordered two months: it was a family disease on his father's side. Having manifested a mischievous disposition to some of his relations, he was continued in the hospital upon the incurable establishment. His temper was naturally violent, and he was easily provoked. As long as he was kept to any employment he conducted himself tolerably well; but when unoccupied, would walk about in a hurried and distracted manner, throwing out the most horrid threats and imprecations. He would often appear to be holding conversations: but these conferences always terminated in a violent quarrel between the imaginary being and himself. He constantly supposed unfriendly people were placed in different parts of the house to torment and annoy him. However violently he might be contesting any subject with these supposed enemies, if directed by the keepers to render them any assistance, he immediately gave up the dispute and went with alacrity. As he got but little sleep, the greatest part of the night was spent in a very noisy and riotous manner. In this state he continued until April 1796, when he was attacked with a paralytic affection, which deprived him of the use of the left side. His articulation was now hardly intelligible; he became childish, got gradually weaker, and died December 28, 1796. He was opened twenty-four hours after death. There was a general opacity of the arachnoid coat, and a small quantity of water between that membrane and the pia mater: the ventricles were much enlarged and contained a considerable quantity of water, by estimation four ounces: the consistence of the brain was natural.

CASE XVII.

M. G. a woman about fifty years of age had been admitted on the incurable establishment in July 1785. She had for some years before been in a disordered state, and was considered as a dangerous patient. Her temper was violent; and if interrupted in her usual habits, she became very furious. Like many others among the incurables, she was an insulated being: she never spoke except when disturbed. Her greatest delight appeared to be in getting into some corner to sleep; and the interval between breakfast and dinner was usually past in this manner. At other times she was generally committing some petty mischief, such as slyly breaking a window, dirtying the rooms of the other patients, or purloining their provisions. She had been for some months in a weak and declining state, but would never give any account of her complaints. On January 5, 1797, she died, apparently worn out. The head was opened three days after death. The pericranium adhered but slightly to the scull, nor was the dura mater firmly attached. There was water between the membranes of the brain; and the want of transparency of the tunica arachnoidea, indicated marks of former inflammation. The posterior part of the hemispheres of the brain was of a brownish colour. In this case there was a considerable appearance of air in the veins; the medullary substance, when cut, was full of bloody points: the lateral ventricles were small, but filled with water: the plexus choroides were loaded with vesicles of a much larger size than usual: the consistence of the brain was natural.

CASE XVIII.

S. T. a woman aged fifty-seven, was admitted into the house January 14, 1797. It was stated by her friends, that she had been disordered eight months: they were unacquainted with any cause, which might have induced the disease. She had evidently suffered a paralytic attack, which considerably affected her speech, and occasioned her to walk lame with the right leg. As she avoided all conversation, it was not possible to collect any further account of her case. Three days after her admission, she had another paralytic stroke, which deprived her entirely of the use of the right side. Two days afterwards she died. She was opened forty-eight hours after death. There was a small quantity of water between the tunica arachnoidea and pia mater, and a number of opake spots on the former membrane. On the pia mater covering the posterior part of the left hemisphere of the brain, there was an extravasated blotch, about the size of a shilling: the medullary substance was unusually loaded with blood: the lateral ventricles were large, but did not contain much water: the consistence of the brain was very soft.

CASE XIX.

W. C. a man aged sixty-three, was admitted into the hospital January 21, 1797. The persons, who attended at his admission, deposed, that he had been disordered five months; that he never had been insane before, and that the disease came on shortly after the death of his son. He was in a very anxious and miserable state. No persuasion could induce him to take nourishment; and it was with extreme difficulty that any food could be forced upon him. He paced about with an hurried step; was often suddenly struck with the idea of having important business to adjust in some distant place, and which would not admit of a moment's delay. Presently after, he would conceive his house to be on fire, and would hastily endeavour to rescue his property from the flames. Then he would fancy that his son was drowning, that he had twice sunk: he was prepared to plunge into the river to save him, as he floated for the last time: every moment appeared an hour until he rose. In this miserable state he continued till the 27th, when, with great perturbation, he suddenly ran into his room, threw himself on the bed, and in a few minutes expired. The head was opened twenty-four hours after death. The pericranium was but slightly adherent to the scull: the tunica arachnoidea, particularly where the hemispheres meet, was of a milky whiteness. Between this membrane, which was somewhat thickened, and the pia mater, there was a very large collection of water: the pia mater was inflamed: the veins of this membrane were enlarged beyond what I had ever before observed: there was a striking appearance of air in the veins: the medullary substance of the brain, when cut into, bled freely, and seemed spungy from the number and enlargement of its vessels: in the ventricles, which were of a natural capacity, there was about half an ounce of water: the brain was of a healthy consistence.

CASE XX.

M. L. a woman aged thirty-eight, was admitted into the house June 11, 1796. From the information of the people who had attended her, it appeared, that she had been disordered six weeks, and that the disease took place shortly after the death of her husband. At the first attack she was violent, but she soon became more calm. She conceived that the overseers of the parish, to which she belonged, meditated her destruction: afterwards she supposed them deeply enamoured of her, and that they were to decide their claims by a battle. During the time she continued in the hospital she was perfectly quiet, although very much deranged. She fancied that a young man, for whom she had formerly entertained a partiality, but who had been dead some years, appeared frequently at her bedside in a state of putrefaction, which left an abominable stench in her room. Soon after she grew suspicious, and became apprehensive of evil intentions in the people about her. She would frequently watch at her door, and, when asked the reason, replied, that she was fully aware of a design, which had been formed, to put her secretly to death. Under the influence of these opinions she continued to her death, which took place on February 8, 1797, in consequence of a violent rheumatic fever. She was opened twelve hours after death. There were two opake spots on the tunica arachnoidea: the pia mater was slightly inflamed: there was a general congestion of blood in the whole contents of the cranium: the consistence of the brain did not differ from what is found in an healthy state.

CASE XXI.

H. C. a woman of about sixty-five years of age, had been admitted on the incurable establishment in the year 1788. I have not been able to collect any particulars of her former history. During the time I had an opportunity of seeing her, she continued in a very violent and irritable state: it was her custom to abuse every one who came near her. The greatest part of the day was passed in cursing the persons she saw about her; and when no one was near, she usually muttered some blasphemy to herself. She died of a fever on February 19, 1797, on the fourth day after the attack. She was opened two days after death. The arachnoid membrane was, in many parts, without its natural transparency: the pia mater was generally suffused with blood, and its vessels were enlarged: the consistence of the brain was firm.

CASE XXII.

J. C. a man aged fifty, was admitted into the hospital August 6, 1796. It was stated that he had been disordered about three weeks, and that the disease had been induced by too great attention to business, and the want of sufficient rest. About four years before, he had been a patient, and was discharged uncured. He was an artful and designing man, and with great ingenuity once effected his escape from the hospital. His time was mostly passed in childish amusements, such as tearing pieces of paper and sticking them on the walls of his room, collecting rubbish and assorting it. However, when he conceived himself unobserved, he was intriguing with other patients, and instructing them in the means, by which, they might escape. Of his disorder he seemed highly sensible, and appeared to approve so much of his confinement, that when his friends wished to have him released, he opposed it, except it should meet with my approbation; telling them, in my presence, that although, he might appear well to them, the medical people of the house, were alone capable of judging of the actual state of his mind; yet I afterwards discovered, that he had instigated them to procure his enlargement, by a relation of the grossest falshoods and unjust complaints. In April 1797, he was permitted to have a month's leave of absence, as he appeared tolerably well, and wished to maintain his family by his industry. For above three weeks of this time, he conducted himself in a very rational and orderly manner. The day preceding that, on which he was to have returned thanks, he appeared gloomy and suspicious, and felt a disinclination for work. The night was passed in a restless manner, but in the morning he seemed better, and proposed coming to the hospital to obtain his discharge. His wife having been absent for a few minutes from the room, found him, on her return, with his throat cut. He was re-admitted as a patient, and expressed great sorrow and penitence for what he had done; and said that it was committed in a moment of rashness and despair. After a long and minute examination, he betrayed nothing incoherent in his discourse. His wound, from which it was stated, that he had lost a large quantity of blood, was attended to by Mr. Crowther, the surgeon to the hospital. Every day he became more dispirited, and at last refused to speak. He died May 29th, about ten days after his re-admission. His head was opened two days after death. There were some slight opacities of the tunica arachnoides, and the pia mater was a little inflamed: the other parts of the brain were in an healthy state, and its consistence natural.

CASE XXIII.

E. L. was a man about seventy-eight years of age; had been admitted on the incurable establishment January 3, 1767. By report, I have understood that he was formerly in the navy, and that his insanity was caused by a disappointment of some promotion which he expected. It was also said that he was troublesome to some persons high in office, which rendered it necessary that he should be confined. At one time he imagined himself to be the king, and insisted on his crown. During the time I had an opportunity of knowing him, he conducted himself in a very gentlemanly manner. His disposition was remarkably placid, and I never remember him to have uttered an unkind or hasty expression. With the other patients he seldom held any conversation. His chief amusement was in reading, and writing letters to the people of the house. Of his books he was by no means choice; he appeared to derive as much amusement from an old catalogue as from the most entertaining performance. His writings always contained directions for his release from confinement; and he never omitted his high titles of God's King, Holy Ghost, Admiral and Physician. He died June 13, 1797, worn out with age. He was opened two days after death. The scull was thick and porous. There was a large quantity of water between the different membranes. The membrana arachnoidea was particularly opake: the veins seemed to contain air: in the medullary substance the vessels were very copious and much enlarged: the lateral ventricles contained two ounces of pellucid water: the consistence of the brain was natural.

It has been stated by a gentleman of great accuracy, and whose situation affords him abundant opportunity of acquiring a knowledge of diseased appearances, that the fluid of hydrocephalus appears to be of the same nature with the water which is found in dropsy of the thorax and abdomen[3]. That this is generally the case, there can be no doubt, from the respectable testimony of the author of the Morbid Anatomy. But in three instances, where I submitted this fluid to experiment, it was incoagulable by acids and by heat: in all of them its consistence was not altered even by boiling. There was, however, a cloudiness produced; and after the liquor had stood some time, a slight deposition took place of animal matter, which, prior to the application of heat or mineral acids, had been dissolved in the fluid. This liquor tinged green the vegetable blues: produced a copious deposition with nitrat of silver, and on evaporation afforded cubic crystals (nitrat of soda). From this examination it was inferred, that the water of the brain, collected in maniacal cases, contained a quantity of uncombined alkali and some common salt. What other substances may enter into its composition, from want of sufficient opportunity, I have not been enabled to determine.

CASE XXIV.

S. W. a woman thirty-five years of age, was admitted into the hospital June 3, 1797. It was stated that she had been one month disordered, and had never experienced any prior affection of the same kind. The disease was said to have been produced by misfortunes which had attended her family, and from frequent quarrels with those who composed it. She was in a truly melancholy state; she was lost to all the comforts of this life, and conceived herself abandoned for ever by God. She refused all food and medicines. In this wretched condition she continued until July 29th, when she lost the use of her right side. On the 30th she became lethargic, and continued so until her death, which happened on August the 3d. She was opened two days after death. There was a large collection of water between the different membranes of the brain, amounting at least to four ounces: the pia mater was very much inflamed, and was separable from the convolutions of the brain with unusual facility: the medullary substance was abundantly loaded with bloody points: the consistence of the brain was remarkably firm.

CASE XXV.

D. W. a man about fifty-eight years of age, had been admitted upon the incurable establishment in 1789. He was of a violent and mischievous disposition, and had nearly killed one of the keepers at a private madhouse, previously to his admission into the hospital. At all times he was equally deranged respecting his opinions, although he was occasionally more quiet and tractable: these intervals were extremely irregular as to their duration and period of return. He was of a very constipated habit, and required large doses of cathartic medicines to procure stools. On August 3, 1797, he was in a very furious state; complained of costiveness, for which he took his ordinary quantity of opening physic, which operated as usual. On the same day he ate his dinner with a good appetite; but about six o'clock in the evening he was struck with hemiplegia, which deprived him completely of the use of his left side. He lay insensible of what passed about him, muttered constantly to himself, and appeared to be keeping up a kind of conversation. The pulse was feeble, but not oppressed or intermitting. He never had any stertor. He continued in this state until the 12th, when he died. He was opened twelve hours after death. There was some water between the tunica arachnoidea and pia mater: the former membrane was opake in many places; bearing the marks of former inflammation: in the veins of the membranes of the brain there was a considerable appearance of air, and they were likewise particularly charged with blood: the vessels of the medullary substance were numerous and enlarged. On opening the right lateral ventricle, which was much distended, it was found filled with dark and grumous blood; some had also escaped into the left, but in quantity inconsiderable when compared with what was contained in the other: the consistence of the brain was very soft.

CASE XXVI.

J. S. a man forty-four years of age, was received into the hospital June 24, 1797. He had been disordered nine months previous to his admission. His insanity was attributed to a violent quarrel, which had taken place with a young woman, to whom he was attached, as he shortly afterwards became sullen and melancholy.

During the time he remained in the house he seldom spoke, and wandered about like a forlorn person. Sometimes he would suddenly stop, and keep his eyes fixed on an object, and continue to stare at it for more than an hour together. Afterwards he became stupid, hung down his head, and drivelled like an ideot. At length he grew feeble and emaciated, his legs were swollen and œdematous, and on September 13th, after eating his dinner, he crawled to his room, where he was found dead about an hour afterwards. He was opened two days after death. The tunica arachnoidea had a milky whiteness, and was thickened. There was a considerable quantity of water between that membrane and the pia mater, which latter was loaded with blood: the lateral ventricles were very much enlarged, and contained, by estimation, about six ounces of transparent fluid: the brain was of its natural consistence.

CASE XXVII.

T. W. a man thirty-eight years of age, was admitted into the house May 16, 1795. He had then been disordered a year. His disease was stated to have arisen, from his having been defrauded, by two of his near relations, of some property, which he had accumulated by servitude. Having remained in the hospital the usual time of trial for cure, he was afterwards continued on the incurable establishment, in consequence of a strong determination he had always shewn, to be revenged on those people who had disposed of his property, and a declared intention of destroying himself. He was in a very miserable state, conceived that he had offended God, and that his soul was burning in Hell. Notwithstanding he was haunted with these dreadful imaginations, he acted with propriety upon most occasions. He took delight in rendering any assistance in his power to the people about the house, and waited on those who were sick, with a kindness that made him generally esteemed. At some period of his life he had acquired an unfortunate propensity to gaming, and whenever he had collected a few pence, he ventured them at cards. His losses were borne with very little philosophy, and the devil was always accused of some unfair interposition.

On September 14, 1797, he appeared jaundiced, the yellowness daily increased, and his depression of mind was more tormenting than ever. From the time he was first attacked by the jaundice he had a strong presentiment that he should die. Although he took the medicines which were ordered, as a mark of attention to those who prescribed them, he was firmly persuaded they could be of no service. The horror and anxiety he felt was, he said, sufficient to kill him independantly of the jaundice.

On the 20th he was drowsy, and on the following day died comatose. He was opened twenty-four hours after death. In some places the tunica arachnoides was slightly opake: the pia mater was inflamed; and in the ventricles were found about two tea-spoonsful of water tinged deeply yellow, and the vesicles of the plexus choroides were of the same colour: in the whole contents of the cranium there was a considerable congestion of blood: the consistence of the brain was natural: the liver was sound: the gallbladder very much thickened, and contained a stone of the mulberry appearance, of a white colour. Another stone was also found in the duodenum.

CASE XXVIII.

R. B. a man sixty-four years of age, was admitted into the hospital September 2, 1797. He had then been disordered three months. It was also stated, that he had suffered an attack of this disease seven years before, which then continued about two months. His disorder had, both times, been occasioned by drinking spirituous liquors to excess. He was a person of liberal education, and had been occasionally employed as usher in a school, and at other times as a librarian and amanuensis. When admitted he was very noisy, and importunately talkative. During the greatest part of the day he was reciting passages from the Greek and Roman poets, or talking of his own literary importance. He became so troublesome to the other madmen, who were sufficiently occupied with their own speculations, that they avoided, and excluded him from the common room; so that he was, at last, reduced to the mortifying situation, of being the sole auditor of his own compositions.

He conceived himself very nearly related to Anacreon, and possessed of the peculiar vein of that poet. He also fancied that he had discovered the longitude, and was very urgent for his liberation from the hospital, that he might claim the reward, to which his discovery was intitled. At length he formed schemes to pay off the national debt: these, however, so much bewildered him that his disorder became more violent than ever, and he was in consequence obliged to be confined to his room. He now, after he had remained two months in the house, was more noisy than before, and got hardly any sleep. These exertions very much reduced him.

In the beginning of January 1798, his conceptions were less distinct, and although his talkativeness continued, he was unable to conclude a single sentence. When he began to speak, his attention was diverted by the first object which caught his eye, or by any sound that struck him. On the 5th he merely muttered; on the 7th he lost the use of his right side, and became stupid and taciturn. In this state he continued until the 14th, when he had another fit; after which, he remained comatose and insensible. On the following day he died. He was opened thirty-six hours after death. The pericranium adhered very loosely to the scull: the tunica arachnoidea was generally opake, and suffused with a brownish hue: a large quantity of water was contained between it and the pia mater: the contents of the cranium were unusually destitute of blood: there was a considerable quantity of water (perhaps four ounces) in the lateral ventricles, which were very much enlarged: the consistence of the brain was very soft.

CASE XXIX.

E. T. a man aged thirty years, was admitted a patient July 23, 1796. The persons who attended related, that he had been disordered eleven months, and that his insanity shortly supervened to a violent fever. It also appeared, from subsequent enquiries, that his mother had been affected with madness.

He was a very violent and mischievous patient, and possessed of great bodily strength and activity. Although confined, he contrived several times during the night to tear up the flooring of his cell; and had also detached the wainscot to a considerable extent, and loosened a number of bricks in the wall. When a new patient was admitted, he generally enticed him into his room, on pretence of being an old acquaintance, and, as soon as he came within his reach, immediately tore his clothes to pieces. He was extremely dexterous with his feet, and frequently took off the hats of those who were near him with his toes, and destroyed them with his teeth. After he had dined he generally bit to pieces a thick wooden bowl, in which his food was served, on the principle of sharpening his teeth against the next meal. He once bit out the testicles of a living cat, because the animal was attached to some person who had offended him. Of his disorder he appeared to be very sensible; and after he had done any mischief, always blamed the keepers for not having secured him so, as to have prevented it. After he had continued a year in the hospital he was retained as an incurable patient. He died February 17, 1798, in consequence of a tumor of the neck. He was opened two days after death. The tunica arachnoides was generally opake, and of a milky whiteness: the vessels of the pia mater were turgid, and its veins contained a quantity of air; about an ounce of water was contained in the lateral ventricles: the consistence of the brain was unusually firm and possessed of considerable elasticity: it is the only instance of this nature which has fallen under my observation.

CHAP. III.

ON THE CAUSES OF INSANITY.

When patients are admitted into Bethlem Hospital, an enquiry is always made of the friends who accompany them, respecting the cause supposed to have occasioned their insanity.

It will readily be conceived that there must be great uncertainty attending the information we are able to procure upon this head: and even from the most accurate accounts, it would be difficult to pronounce, that the circumstances which are related to us have actually produced the effect. The friends and relatives of patients are, upon many occasions, very delicate upon this point, and cautious of exposing their frailties or immoral habits: and when the disease is a family one, they are oftentimes still more reserved in disclosing the truth.

Fully aware of the incorrect statement frequently made concerning these causes,

I have been at no inconsiderable pains to correct or confirm the first information, by subsequent enquiries.

The causes which I have been enabled most certainly to ascertain, may be divided into *physical* and *moral*.

Under the first are comprehended *repeated intoxication*; *blows* received upon the head; fever, particularly when accompanied with delirium; mercury largely or injudiciously administered; the suppression of periodical or occasional discharges and secretions; hereditary disposition, and paralytic affections.

By the second class of causes, which I have termed *moral*, are meant those which are applied directly to the mind. Such are the long endurance of grief, ardent and ungratified desires, religious terror, the disappointment of pride, sudden fright, fits of anger, prosperity humbled by misfortunes[4]: in short, the frequent and uncurbed indulgence of any passion or emotion, and any sudden and violent affection of the mind.

There are, doubtless, many other causes of both classes which may tend to produce the disease. Those which have been stated are such as I am most familiar with; or, to speak more accurately, such are the circumstances most generally found to have preceded this affection.

The greatest number of these moral causes may, perhaps, be traced to the errors of education, which often plant in the youthful mind those seeds of madness, which the slightest circumstances readily awaken into growth.

It should be as much the object of teachers of youth, to subjugate the passions, as to discipline the intellect. The tender mind should be prepared to expect the natural and certain effects of causes: its propensity to indulge an avaricious thirst for that which is unattainable should be quenched: nor should it be suffered to acquire a fixed and invincible attachment to that which is fleeting and perishable.

Of the more immediate, or, as it is generally termed, the proximate cause of this disease, I profess to know nothing. Whenever the functions of the brain shall be fully understood, and the use of its different parts ascertained, we may then be enabled to judge, how far disease, attacking any of these parts, may increase, diminish, or otherwise alter its functions. But this appears a degree of knowledge which we are not likely soon to attain. It seems, however, not improbable that the only source from whence the most copious and certain information can be drawn, is a laborious attention to the particular appearances which morbid states of this organ may present.

From the preceding dissections of insane persons, it may be inferred, that madness has always been connected with disease of the brain, and of its membranes. These cases have not been selected from a variety of others, but comprize the entire number which have fallen under my observation. Having no particular theory to build up, they have been related purely for the advancement of science and of truth.

It may be a matter affording much diversity of opinion, whether these morbid appearances of the brain be the cause or the effect of madness: it may be observed, that they have been found in all states of the disease. When the brain has been injured from external violence, its functions have been generally impaired if inflammation of its substance, or more delicate membranes has ensued. The same appearances have for the most part been detected when patients have died of phrenitis, or in the delirium of fever: in these instances the derangement of the intellectual functions appears evidently to have been caused by the inflammation. If in mania the same appearances be found, there will be no necessity of calling in the aid of other causes to account for the effect; indeed it would be difficult to discover them. Those who entertain an opposite opinion, are obliged to suppose, *a disease of the mind*. Such a morbid affection, from the limited nature of my powers, perhaps I have never been able to conceive. Possessing, however, little knowledge of metaphysical controversy, I shall only offer a few remarks upon this part of the subject, and beg pardon for having at all touched it.

Perhaps it is not more difficult to suppose that matter peculiarly arranged may *think*, than to conceive the union of an immaterial being with a corporeal substance. It is questioning the infinite wisdom and power of the Deity to say, that he does not, or cannot arrange and organize matter so that it shall think. When we find insanity, as far as has hitherto been observed, uniformly accompanied with disease of the brain, is it not more just to conclude, that such organic affection has produced this incorrect association of ideas, than that a being, which is immaterial, incorruptible and immortal, should be subject to the gross and subordinate changes which matter necessarily undergoes?

But let us imagine *a disease of ideas*. In what manner are we to effect a cure? To this subtle spirit the doctor can apply no medicines. But though so refined as to elude the force of material remedies, some may however think that it may be reasoned with. The good effects which have resulted from exhibiting logic as a remedy for madness, must be sufficiently known to every one who has conversed with insane persons, and must be considered as time very judiciously employed: speaking more gravely, it will readily be acknowledged, by persons acquainted with this disease, that if insanity be a disease of ideas, we possess no corporeal remedies for it: and that to endeavour to convince madmen of their errors, by reasoning, is folly in those who attempt it, since there is always in madness the firmest conviction of the truth of what is false, and which the clearest and most circumstantial evidence cannot remove.

ON THE PROBABLE EVENT OF THE DISEASE.

The prediction of the event in cases of insanity must be the result of accurate and extensive experience; and even then it will be a matter of very great uncertainty. The practitioner can only be led to suppose that patients of a particular description will recover, from knowing, that under the same circumstances, a certain number have been actually restored to health.

The practice of an individual, however active and industrious he may be, is insufficient to accumulate a stock of facts, necessary to form the ground of a regular and correct prognosis: it is therefore to be wished, that those who exclusively confine themselves to this department of the profession, would occasionally communicate to the world the result of their observations. Physicians attending generally to diseases, have not reserved in imparting to the public the amount of their labours and success; but with regard to this disorder, those who have devoted their whole attention to its treatment have either been negligent or cautious of giving information respecting it. Whenever the powers of the mind are concentrated to one object, we may naturally expect a more rapid progress in the attainment of knowledge; we have therefore only to lament the want of observations upon this subject, and endeavour to repair it. The records of Bethlem Hospital have afforded me some satisfactory information, though far from the whole of what I wished to obtain. From them and my own observations the prognosis of this disease is, with great diffidence, submitted to the reader.

In our own climate women are more frequently affected with insanity than men. Several persons who superintend private mad-houses have assured me, that the number of females brought in annually considerably exceeds that of the males. From the year 1748, to 1794, comprizing a period of forty-six years, there have been admitted into Bethlem

Hospital 4832 women, and 4042 men. The natural processes which women undergo, of menstruation, parturition, and of preparing nutriment for the infant, together with the diseases to which they are subject at these periods, and which are frequently remote causes of insanity, may, perhaps, serve to explain their greater disposition to this malady. As to the proportion in which they recover, compared with males, it may be stated, that of 4832 women affected, 1402 were discharged cured; and that of the 4042 men, 1155 recovered. It is proper here to mention that in general we know but little of what becomes of those who are discharged, a certain number of those cured occasionally relapse; and some of those who are discharged uncured afterwards recover: perhaps in the majority of instances, where they relapse, they are sent back to Bethlem. To give some idea of the number so readmitted, it may be mentioned, that, during the last two years, there have been admitted 389 patients, 53 of whom had at some former time been in the house. There are such a variety of circumstances, which, supposing they did relapse, might prevent them from returning, that it can only be stated, with confidence, that within twelve months (the time allowed as a trial of cure) so many have been discharged perfectly well.

To shew how frequently insanity supervenes on parturition, it may be remarked, that, from the year 1784 to 1794 inclusive, 80 patients have been admitted, whose disorder shortly followed the puerperal state. Women affected from this cause recover in a larger proportion than patients of any other description of the same age. Of these 80, 50 have perfectly recovered. The first symptom of the approach of this disease, after delivery, is want of sleep; the milk is afterwards secreted in less quantity, and, when the mind becomes more violently disordered, it is totally suppressed.

From whatever cause this disease may be produced in women, it is considered as very unfavourable to recovery, if they are worse at the period of menstruation, or have their catamenia in very small or immoderate quantities.

At the first attack of the disease, and for some months afterwards, during its continuance, females most commonly labour under amenorrhœa. The natural and healthy return of this discharge generally precedes convalescence.

From the following statement it will be seen, that insane persons recover in proportion to their youth, and that as they advance in years, the disease is less frequently cured. It comprizes a period of about ten years, viz. from 1784 to 1794. In the first column the age is noticed, in the second the number of patients admitted; the third contains the number cured; the fourth those who were discharged not cured.

Age between	Number admitted.	Number discharged cured.	Number discharged uncured.
10 and 20	113	78	35
20 and 30	488	200	288
30 and 40	527	180	347
40 and 50	362	87	275
50 and 60	143	25	118
60 and 70	31	4	27
	1664	574	1090
	Total admitted.	Total cured.	Total uncured.

From this table it will be seen, that when the disease attacks persons advanced in life, the prospect of recovery is but small.

From the very rare instances of complete cure, or durable amendment, among the class of patients deemed incurable, as well as from the infrequent recovery of those who have been admitted, after the complaint has been of more than twelve months standing, I am led to conclude, that the chance of cure is less, in proportion to the length of time which the disorder shall have continued.

Although patients, who have been affected with insanity more than a year, are not admissible into the hospital, to continue there for the usual time of trial for cure, namely, a twelvemonth, yet, at the discretion of the committee, they may be received into it from Lady-day to Michaelmas, at which latter period they are removed. In the course of the last ten years, fifty-six patients of this description have been received, of whom only one has been discharged cured. This patient, who was a woman, has since relapsed twice, and is, at present, in the hospital.

When the reader contrasts the preceding statement with the account recorded in the report of the committee, appointed to examine the physicians who have attended his majesty, &c. he will either be inclined to deplore the unskilfulness or mismanagement which has prevailed among those medical persons who have directed the treatment of mania in the largest public institution, in this kingdom, of its kind, compared with the success which has attended the private practice of an individual; or, *to require some other evidence, than the bare assertions of the man pretending to have performed such cures*[5]. It was deposed by that reverend and celebrated physician, that of patients placed under his care within three months after the attack of the disease, nine out of ten had recovered[6]; and also that the age was of no signification, unless the patient had been afflicted before with the same malady[7].

How little soever I might be disposed to doubt such a bold, unprecedented, and marvellous account, yet, I must acknowledge, that my mind would have been much more satisfied as to the truth of that assertion, had it been plausibly made out, or had the circumstances been otherwise than feebly recollected by that very successful practitioner. Medicine has generally been esteemed a progressive science, in which its professors have confessed themselves indebted to great preparatory study, and long subsequent experience, for the knowledge they have acquired; but in the case to which we are now alluding, the outset of the doctor's practice was marked with such splendid success, that time and observation have been unable to increase it.

This astonishing number of cures has been effected by the vigorous agency of remedies, which others have not hitherto been so fortunate as to discover; by remedies which, when remote causes have been operating for twenty-seven years, such as weighty business, severe exercise, too great abstemiousness and little rest, are possessed of adequate power directly to *meet and counteract* such causes[8].

It will be seen by the table that a greater number of patients have been admitted between the age of thirty and forty, than during any other equal period of life. There may be some reasons assigned for the increased proportion of insane persons at this age.

Although I have made no exact calculation, yet, from a great number of cases, it appears to be the time, when the hereditary disposition is most frequently called into action; or, to speak more plainly, it is that stage of life when persons, whose families have been insane, are most liable to become mad. If it can be made to appear, that at this period people are more subject to be acted upon by the remote causes of the disease, or that a greater number of such causes are then applied, we may be enabled satisfactorily to explain it. At this age people are generally established in their different occupations, are married, and have families; their habits are more strongly formed, and the interruptions of them are, consequently, attended with greater anxiety and regret. Under these circumstances, they feel the misfortunes of life more exquisitely. Adversity does not depress the individual for himself alone, but as involving his partner and his offspring in wretchedness and ruin. In youth, we feel desirous only of present good; at the middle age, we become more provident and anxious for the future; the mind assumes a serious character, and religion, as it is justly or improperly impressed, imparts comfort, or excites apprehension and terror.

By misfortunes the habits of intoxication are readily formed. Those, who in their youth have shaken off calamity as a superficial incumbrance, at the middle age feel it corrode and penetrate: and when fermented liquors have once dispelled the gloom of despondency, and taught the mind either to excite a temporary assemblage of cheerful scenes, or to disdain the terror of impending misery, it is natural to recur to the same, though destructive cause, to reproduce the effect.

Patients, who are in a furious state, recover in a larger proportion than those who are depressed and melancholick. An hundred violent, and the same number of melancholick cases were selected. Of the former, sixty-two were discharged well; of the latter, only twenty-seven. When the furious state is succeeded by melancholy, and after this shall have continued a short time, the violent paroxysm returns, the hope of recovery is very slight. Indeed, whenever these states of the disease frequently change, such alternation may be considered as unfavourable.

Where the complaint has been induced from remote physical causes, the proportion of those who recover is considerably greater, than where it has arisen from causes of a moral nature. In those instances where insanity has been produced by a train of unavoidable misfortunes, as where the father of a large family, with the most laborious exertions, ineffectually struggles to maintain it, the number who recover is very small indeed.

Paralytic affections are a much more frequent cause of insanity than has been commonly supposed. In those affected from this cause, we are, on enquiry, enabled to trace a sudden affection, or fit, to have preceded the disease. These patients usually bear marks of such affection, independent of their insanity: the speech is impeded, and the mouth drawn aside; an arm, or leg, is more or less deprived of its capacity of being moved by the will: and in by far the greatest number of these cases the memory is particularly affected. Very few of these cases have received any benefit in the hospital; and from the enquiries I have been able to make at the private houses, where they have been afterwards confined, it has appeared, that they have either died suddenly from apoplexy, or have had repeated fits, from the effects of which they have sunk into a stupid state, and have gradually dwindled away.

When the natural small-pox attacks insane persons, it most commonly proves fatal.

When insanity supervenes on epilepsy, of where the latter disease is induced by insanity, a cure is very seldom effected: from my own observation, I do not recollect a single case of recovery.

When patients during their convalescence become more corpulent than they were before, it is a favourable symptom; and, as far as I have remarked, such persons have very seldom relapsed.

METHOD OF CURE.

This part of the subject may be divided into management, and treatment by medicine.

As most men perceive the faults of others without being aware of their own, so insane people easily detect the nonsense of other madmen without being able to discover, or even to be made sensible of the incorrect associations of their own ideas. For this reason it is highly important, that he who pretends to regulate the conduct of such patients, should first have learned the management of himself. It should be the great object of the superintendant to gain the confidence of the patient, and to awaken in him respect and obedience: but it will readily be seen, that such confidence, obedience, and respect, can only be procured by superiority of talents, discipline of temper, and dignity of manners. Imbecility, misconduct, and empty consequence, although enforced with the most tyrannical severity, may excite fear, but this will always be mingled with contempt.

In speaking of the management of insane persons, it is to be understood that the superintendant must first obtain an ascendency over them. When this is once effected, he will be enabled, on future occasions, to direct and regulate their conduct, according as his better judgment may suggest. He should possess firmness; and, when occasion may require, should exercise his authority in a peremptory manner. He should never threaten, but execute: and when the patient has misbehaved, should confine him immediately. As example operates more forcibly than precept, I have found it useful, to order the delinquent to be confined in the presence of the other patients. It displays authority; and the person who has misbehaved becomes awed by the spectators, and more readily submits. It also prevents the wanton exercise of force, and those cruel and unmanly advantages which might be taken when the patient and keeper are shut up in a private room. When the patient is vigorous and powerful, two, or more should assist in securing him; by these means it will be easily effected; for, where the force of the contending persons is nearly equal, the mastery cannot be obtained without difficulty and danger.

As management is employed to produce a salutary change upon the patient, and to restrain him from committing violence on others and himself, it may be proper here to enquire, upon what occasions, and to what extent, coercion may be used. The term coercion has generally been understood in a very formidable sense, and not without reason. It has been recommended, by very high medical authority, to inflict corporal punishment upon maniacs, with a view of rendering them rational by impressing terror[9]. What success may have followed such disgraceful and inhuman treatment I have not yet learned, nor should I be desirous of meeting with any one who could give me the information. If the patient be so far deprived of understanding, as to be insensible why he is punished, such correction, setting aside its cruelty, is manifestly absurd. And if his state be such, as to be conscious of the impropriety of his conduct, there are other methods more mild and effectual.

Would any rational practitioner, in a case of phrenitis, or in the delirium of fever, order his patient to be scourged? He would rather suppose that the brain or its membranes were inflamed, and that the incoherence of discourse, and violence of action, were produced by such local disease. We have seen, by the preceding dissections, that the contents of the cranium, in all the instances that have occurred to me, have been in a morbid state. It should therefore be the object of the practitioner to remove such disease, rather than irritate and torment the sufferer. Coercion should only be considered as a protesting and salutary restraint.

In the most violent state of the disease, the patient should be kept alone in a dark and quiet room, so that he may not be affected by the stimuli of light or sound, such abstraction more readily disposing to sleep. As in this violent state there is a strong propensity to associate ideas, it is particularly important to prevent the accession of such as might be transmitted through the medium of the senses. The hands should be properly secured, and the patient should also be confined by one leg: this will prevent him from committing any violence. The straight waistcoat is admirably calculated to prevent patients from doing mischief to themselves; but in the furious state, and particularly in warm weather, it irritates and increases that restlessness, which patients of this description usually labour under. They then scorn the incumbrance of cloathing, and seem to delight in exposing their bodies to the atmosphere. Where the patient is in a condition to be sensible of restraint, he may be punished for improper behaviour by confining him to his room, by degrading him, and not allowing him to associate with the convalescents, and by withholding certain indulgences he had been accustomed to enjoy.

As madmen frequently entertain very high, and even romantic notions of honour, they are rendered much more tractable by wounding their pride, than by severity of discipline.

Speaking of the effects of management on a very extensive scale, I can truly declare, that by gentleness of manner, and kindness of treatment, I have never failed to obtain the confidence, and conciliate the esteem of insane persons, and have succeeded by these means in procuring from them respect and obedience. There are certainly some patients who are not to be trusted, and in whom malevolence forms the prominent feature of their character: such persons should always be kept under a certain restraint, but this is not incompatible with kindness and humanity.

Considering how much we are the creatures of habit, it might naturally be hoped, and experience justifies the expectation, that madmen might be benefited by bringing their actions into a system of regularity. It might be supposed, that as thought precedes action, that whenever the ideas are incoherent, the actions will also be irregular. Most probably they would be so if uncontrouled; but custom, confirmed into habit, destroys this natural propensity, and renders them correct in their behaviour, though they still remain equally depraved in their intellects.

We have a number of patients in Bethlem Hospital whose ideas are in the most disordered state, who yet act, upon ordinary occasions, with great steadiness and propriety, and are capable of being trusted to a considerable extent. A fact of such importance in the history of the human mind, might lead us to hope, that by superinducing different habits of thinking, the irregular associations may be corrected.

It is impossible to effect this suddenly, or by reasoning, for madmen can never be convinced of the folly of their opinions. Their belief in them is firmly fixed, and cannot be shaken. The more frequently these opinions are recurred to under a conviction of their truth, the deeper they subside in the mind and become more obstinately entangled: the object should therefore be to prevent such recurrence by occupying the mind on different subjects, and thus diverting it from the favorite and accustomed train of ideas. As I have been induced to suppose, from the appearances on dissection, that the immediate cause of this disease probably consists in a morbid affection of the brain, all modes of cure by reasoning, or conducting the current of thought into different channels, must be ineffectual, so long as such local disease shall continue. It is, however, likely that insanity is often continued by habit; that incoherent associations, frequently recurred to, become received as truths, in the same manner as a tale, which, although untrue, by being repeatedly told, shall be credited at last by the narrator, as if it had certainly happened. It should likewise be observed, that these incorrect associations of ideas are acquired in the same way as just ones are formed, and that such are as likely to remain, as the most accurate opinions. The generality of minds are very little capable of tracing the origin of their ideas; there are many opinions we are in possession of, with the history and acquisition of which, we are totally unacquainted. We see this in a remarkable manner in patients who are recovering: they will often say such appearances have been presented to my mind with all the force and reality of truth: I saw them as plainly as I now behold any other object, and can hardly be persuaded that they did not occur. It also does not unfrequently happen, that patients will declare, that certain notions are forced into their minds, of which they see the folly and incongruity, and complain that they cannot prevent their intrusion.

It is of great service to establish a system of regularity in the actions of insane people. They should be made to rise, take exercise, and food, at stated times. Independently of such regularity contributing to health, it also renders them much more easily manageable.

As the patient should be taught to view the superintendant as a superior person, the latter should be particularly cautious never to deceive him. Madmen are generally more hurt at deception than punishment; and whenever they detect the imposition, never fail to lose that confidence and respect, which they ought to entertain for the person who governs them.

Confinement is always necessary in cases of insanity, and should be enforced as early in the complaint as possible. By confinement, it is to be understood that the patient should be removed from home. During his continuance at his own house he can never be kept in a tranquil state. The interruptions of his family, the loss of the accustomed obedience of his servants, and the idea of being under restraint in a place where he considers himself the master, will be constant sources of irritation to his mind. It is also known, from considerable experience, that of those patients who have remained under the immediate care of their relatives and friends, very few have recovered. Even the visits of their friends, when they are violently disordered, are productive of great inconvenience, as they are always more unquiet and ungovernable for some time afterwards. It is a well-known fact, that they are less disposed to acquire a dislike to those who are strangers, than to those with whom they have been intimately acquainted; they become therefore less dangerous, and are more easily restrained.

It frequently happens, that patients who have been brought immediately from their families, and who have been said to be in a violent and ferocious state, become suddenly calm and tractable, when placed in the hospital. On the other hand, it is equally certain, that there are many patients, who have for a length of time conducted themselves in a very orderly manner under confinement, whose disorder speedily recurs after being suffered to return to their families. When they are in a convalescent state, the occasional visits of their friends are attended with manifest advantage. Such an intercourse imparts consolation, and presents views of future happiness and comfort.

Many patients have received considerable benefit by change of situation, and this sometimes takes place very shortly after the removal. In what particular cases, or stages of the disease, this may be recommended, I am not enabled by sufficient experience to determine.

MEDICINE.

It is only intended, in this part of the subject, to speak of those medicines which I have administered, by the direction of Dr. Monro, the present celebrated and judicious physician to Bethlem Hospital, (to whom I gratefully acknowledge many and serious obligations) without descending to a minute detail of the hospital practice, or of the order in which they are commonly exhibited. Of the effects of such remedies, I am able to speak with considerable confidence, as they have come immediately under my own observation.

Bleeding.—Where the patient is strong and of a plethoric habit, and where the disorder has not been of any long continuance, bleeding has been found of considerable advantage, and, as far as I have yet observed, is the most beneficial remedy that has been employed. The melancholic cases have been equally relieved with the maniacal by this mode of treatment. Venesection by the arm is, however, inferior in its goods effects to blood taken from the head by cupping. This operation, performed in the manner to which I have been accustomed, consists in having the head previously shaven, and six or eight cupping glasses applied on the scalp; By these means any quantity of blood may be taken, and in as short a time, as by an orifice made in a vein by the lancet. When the raving paroxysm has continued for a considerable time, and the scalp has become unusually flaccid; or where a stupid state has succeeded to violence of considerable duration, no benefit has been derived from bleeding; indeed these states are generally attended by a degree of bodily weakness, sufficient to prohibit such practice independently of other considerations.

The quantity of blood to be taken, must be left to the discretion of the practitioner: from eight to sixteen ounces may be drawn, and the operation occasionally repeated, as circumstances may require.

In the few cases where blood was drawn at the commencement of the disease from the arm, and from patients who were extremely furious and ungovernable, it was covered with a buffy coat; but in other cases it has seldom or never such an appearance. In more than two hundred patients, male and female, who were let blood by venesection, there were only six, whose blood could be termed sizy.

In some few instances hemoptysis has preceded convalescence, as has also a bleeding from, the hemorrhoidal veins. Epistaxis has not, to my knowledge, ever occurred.

Purging. — An opinion has long prevailed, that mad people are particularly constipated, and likewise extremely difficult to be purged. From all the observations I have been able to make, insane patients, on the contrary, are of very delicate and irritable bowels, and are well and copiously purged by a common cathartic draught. That which is commonly employed in the hospital is prepared agreeably to the following formula.

℞. Infusi sennæ ʒiss ad ʒij.

Tincturæ sennæ ʒi ad ʒij.

Syrupi spinæ cervinæ ʒi ad ʒij.

This seldom fails of procuring four or five stools, and frequently a greater number.

In confirmation of what I have advanced respecting the irritable state of intestines in mad people, it may be mentioned, that the ordinary complaints with which they are affected, are diarrhœa and dysentery: these are sometimes very violent and obstinate.

Diarrhœa very often proves a natural cure of insanity; at least there is every reason to suppose that such evacuation has frequently very much contributed to it. The number of cases which might be adduced in confirmation of this observation is considerable, and the speedy convalescence after such evacuation is still more remarkable.

In many cases of insanity there prevails a great degree of insensibility, so that patients have appeared hardly to feel the passing of setons, the application of blisters, or the operation of cupping. On many occasions I have known the urine retained for a considerable time, without the patient complaining of any pain, though it is well known that there is no affection more distressing than distention of the bladder. Of this general insensibility the intestinal canal may be supposed to partake: but this is not commonly the case, and if it should, would be widely different from a particular and exclusive torpor of the primæ viæ.

There are some circumstances unconnected with disease of mind, which might dispose insane persons to costiveness. I now speak of such as are confined, and who come more directly under our observation. When they are mischievously disposed, they require a greater degree of restraint, and are consequently deprived of that air and exercise, which so much contributes to regularity of bowels. It is well known, that those who have been in the habits of free living, and who come suddenly to a more spare diet, are very much disposed to costiveness. But to adduce the fairest proof of what has been advanced, I can truly state, that incurable patients, who have for many years been confined in the house, are subject to no inconveniences from constipation. Many patients are averse to food, and where little is taken in, the egesta must be inconsiderable.

To return from this degression: it is concluded, from very ample experience, that cathartic medicines are of the greatest service, and ought to be considered as an indispensable remedy in cases of insanity. The good sense and experience of every practitioner must direct him as to the dose, and frequency, with which these remedies are to be employed, and of the occasions where they would be prejudicial.

Vomiting.—However strongly this practice may have been recommended, and how much soever it may at present prevail, I am sorry that it is not in my power to speak of it favourably. In many instances, and in some where blood-letting has been previously employed, paralytic affections have within a few hours supervened on the exhibition of an emetic, more especially where the patient has been of a full habit, and has had the appearance of an increased determination to the head.

It has been for many years the practice of Bethlem Hospital, to administer to the curable patients four or five emetics in the spring of the year; but, on consulting my book of cases, I have not found that patients have been particularly benefited by the use of this remedy. From one grain and half to two grains of tartarized antimony has been the usual dose, which has hardly ever failed of procuring full vomiting. In the few instances where the plan of exhibiting this medicine in nauseating doses was pursued for a considerable time, it by no means answered the expectations, which, by very high authority, had been raised in its favour. Where the tartarized antimony, given with this intention, operated as a purgative, it generally produced beneficial effects.

Camphor. — This remedy has been highly extolled, and doubtless with reason, by those who have recommended it. My own experience merely extends to ten cases, a number from which no decisive inference of its utility ought to be drawn. The dose was gradually increased from five grains to two drams twice a day; and in nine cases the use of this remedy was continued for the space of two months. Of the patients, to whom the camphor was given, only two recovered: one of these had no symptoms of convalescence for several months after the use of this remedy had been abandoned; the other, a melancholick patient, certainly mended during the time he was taking it; but he was never able to bear more than ten grains thrice a day. He complained that it made him feel as if he was intoxicated.

Cold Bathing.—This remedy having for the most part been employed in conjunction with others, it becomes difficult to ascertain how far it may be exclusively beneficial in this disease. The instances where it has been separately used for the cure of insanity, are too few to enable me to draw any satisfactory conclusions. I may, however, safely relate, that, in many instances, paralytic affections have in a few hours supervened on cold bathing, especially where the patient has been in a furious state, and of a plethoric habit: in some of these cases vertigo has been induced, and in others a considerable degree of fever. If I might be permitted to give an opinion on this subject, the benefit principally derived from this remedy has been in the latter stages of the disease, and when the system had been previously lowered by evacuations.

Blisters have in several cases been applied to the head, and a very copious discharge maintained for many days, but without any manifest advantage. The late Dr. John Monro, who had, perhaps, seen more cases of this disease than any other practitioner, and who, joined to his extensive experience, possessed the talent of accurate observation, mentions, that he "never saw the least good effect of blisters in madness, unless it was at the beginning while there was some degree of fever, or when they have been applied to particular symptoms accompanying this complaint[10]."

In a few cases setons have been employed, but no benefit has been derived from their use, although the discharge was continued above two months.

Respecting opium, it may be observed, that whenever it has been exhibited during a violent paroxysm, it has hardly ever procured sleep; but, on the contrary, has rendered those who have taken it much more furious: and, where it has for a short time produced rest, the patient has, after its operation, awoke in a state of increased violence.

FINIS.

Footnotes:

[1] This gritty matter, subjected to chemical examination, was found to be *phosphat of lime*.

[2] This appearance I have found frequently to occur in maniacs who have suffered a violent paroxysm of considerable duration: and in such cases, when there has been an opportunity of inspecting the contents of the cranium after death, water has been found between the dura mater and arachnoid membrane.

[3] Morbid Anatomy, page 304.

[4]

" — —Nessun   maggior   dolore,
"Che   ricordarsi   del   tempo   felice
"Nella   miseria."
Dante.

[5] Vide Report, Part 2d, p. 25.

[6] Report, p. 59.

[7] Ibid. 57.

[8] Report, p. 54.

[9] Vide Cullen, first lines, vol. iv. p. 154.

[10] Vide Remarks on Dr. Battie's Treatise on Madness.